# DISPENSE -SATION

A Pharmacist's Rx for a

## Laugh!

Date

MD
Signature

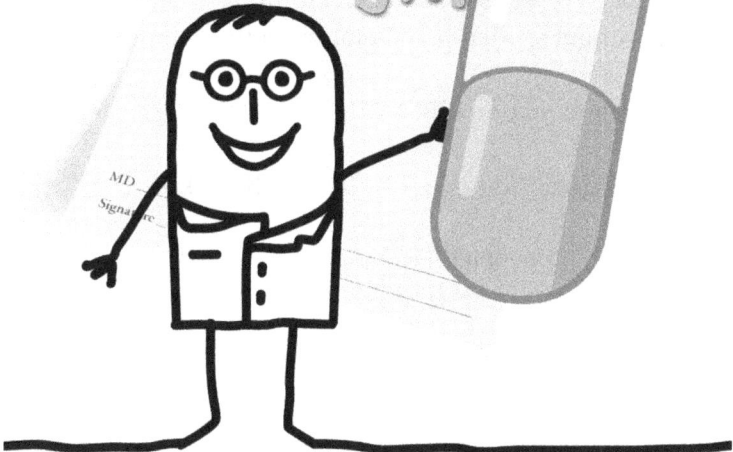

Christopher Holl

**Dispense-sation**
**A Pharmacist's Rx for a Laugh!**
**Christopher Holl**

Published by A.J. Neal Publishing
P.O. Box 1469
Jackson, NJ 08527

Cover and Interior Design KarrieRoss.com
Copyediting by Lynette M. Smith

Print edition ISBN: 978-0-9851442-2-7

Electronic edition ISBN: 978-0-9851442-4-1

First Printing 2014

Library of Congress Control Number: 201491593

*To my mother*

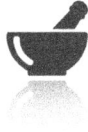

Always laugh when you can,
it is cheap medicine.
–*George Gordon Byron*

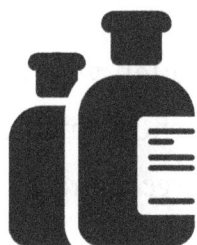

# Contents

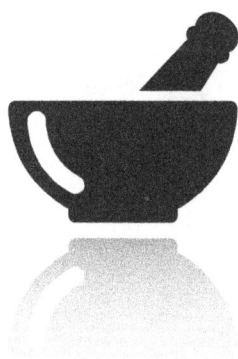

# Introduction

Who am I to publish a book that has anything to do with you, the retail pharmacist, and your profession? I was born to non-pharmacist parents, didn't take organic chemistry in college, never worked in a pharmacy and married a non-pharmacist wife. I am an industry partner, though, and during the past 14 years have spoken with thousands of you in the field, during advisory meetings and at medical conventions.

I've sat for countless hours in research, all across the country, listening to you. You've shared your knowledge, insights on new products, patient interactions and perspectives on potential marketing campaigns. Mostly, you've shared yourselves, and what it's like to be a pharmacist today. I've gained a sense of what frustrates you as well as what you find satisfying. It's clear to me that whether you've been practicing for three years or thirty, at the end of the (long!) day, what keeps you going as a community pharmacist is your desire to help patients and make a difference in their lives.

It's becoming more challenging to do that in a retail environment, as the labyrinthine health care system makes ever increasing demands on you. You are being pulled in dozens of directions. Workload is heavier and faster. Daily dealings with managed (*don't*) care, "the suits" at corporate, patients with no patience, the "McPharmacy atmosphere"… and the list goes on. Seems like everyone wants "a piece of you," so not surprisingly, no one is suggesting you get off your feet, take a break and catch your breath.

Until now. That's why I created *Dispense-sation*. You *do* deserve a break, and this book says it's okay to take one… and have a few laughs too!

My hope is that some humor will provide a brief "mental vacation" and help recharge your batteries. Therefore, this book is a collection of family-friendly jokes culled from the public domain and organized by topics you'll find relevant to your work. In some cases, the humor has been tweaked to be more "pharmacist-centric." Additionally, I've compiled material gathered and shared by some of your fellow pharmacists in their websites and blogs. There are no "sacred cows" regarding who gets poked fun at. Although not everything you deal with on a daily basis is included, an attempt has been made to ensure the most memorable is!

Additionally, the chapter, "Famous Pharmacists," celebrates a few distinguished pharmacists and their important contributions to our world.

Hopefully, this all works in an entertaining way to recognize and appreciate you and affirm your chosen profession.

Now, sit back, relax and have a few laughs (unless it's Monday!)

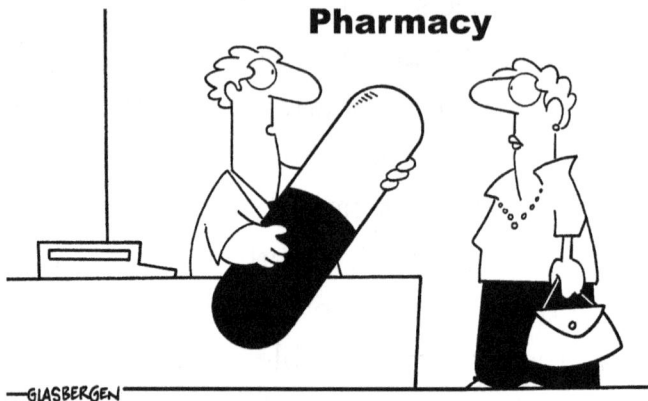

**Pharmacy**

—GLASBERGEN—

"Each capsule contains your medication,
plus a treatment for each of its side effects."

# 2

# No Laughing Matter?

When you're busy filling nearly 4,000,000,000 (yes, four billion!) prescriptions per year, it's hard to do much of anything else, let alone find time to laugh or something to laugh at. But, let's not forget what *Reader's Digest* says— that "laughter is the best medicine" for whatever troubles us. So, here are a few jokes with you in mind, in case there's anything on your mind. It's one medicine you *don't* have to fill!

TWO WOMEN, out for a walk, came upon a frog who said, "Pick me up and kiss me and I'll turn back into a hardworking, honest and highly educated pharmacist." The first woman picked up the frog and put him in her purse. The second asked, "Why not kiss him?" She replied, "Hardworking, honest and highly educated pharmacists are pretty common nowadays—but a talking frog, now that's something!"

A doctor jots down notes for a speech he is giving at the local AMA dinner. Unfortunately, when he stands in front of his colleagues later that night, he can't read his writing. So he asks, "Is there a pharmacist in the house?"

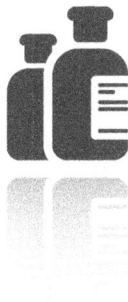

AS A PROVIDER in a recently formed accountable care organization, a pharmacist visits a nursing home to review the medications of its residents. Sitting with an elderly patient, he notices a bowl of peanuts beside her bed and takes one. As they talk, he can't help himself and eats one after another. By the time they are through talking, the bowl is empty. He says, "Ma'am, I'm sorry, but I seem to have eaten all of your peanuts." "That's okay," she says, "they would have just sat there. Without my teeth, all I can do is suck the chocolate off and put them back!"

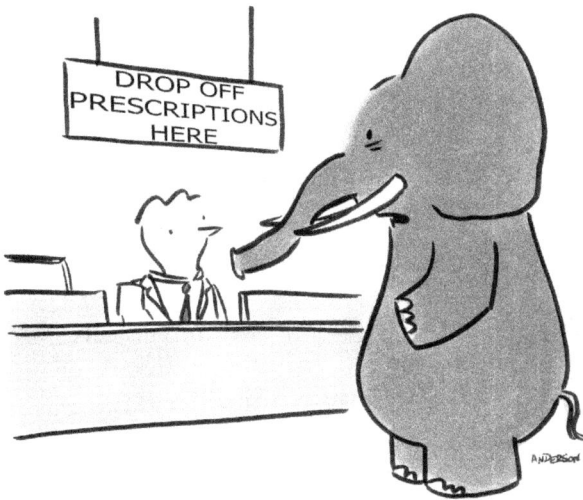

"I need the best antihistamine you have."

A VERY BUSY, hard-working, independent pharmacist was spending a rare, quiet weekend at home with his family. A problem developed with the kitchen and bathroom sinks, so he called a plumber. The plumber assessed the situation and told the pharmacist, "I can fix the problem, but it's double time on weekends—$80 per hour!" "Eighty dollars per hour!" he exclaimed. "Why, I'm a pharmacy owner and that's more than I make!" "Hey, don't feel bad," said the plumber. "When I owned a pharmacy, I didn't make that much, either."

Lady says to pharmacist: "Why does my prescription medication have 40 side effects?" Pharmacist replies: "Because that's all we've documented so far."

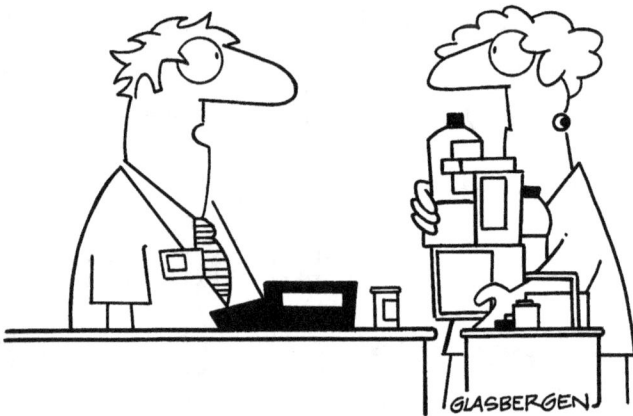

**PHARMACY**

"Coming in for your prescription and buying a ton of other stuff you really don't need ...that's one of the side effects."

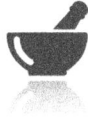

# 3

# You Know You're a Pharmacist When…

When I was a child, whenever my Great Aunt Marie treated us to a donut, she would kid us by saying, "I'll eat the donut, and you can have the hole." Ah, yes, *the donut hole*. A reason to laugh in my childhood is now symbolic of yet another complexity for the retail pharmacist. But you regularly handle these matters with aplomb and at times with humor, as evidenced by some barbs you've shared about "knowing" what's it's like to be a pharmacist.

When you decide to either eat or go
to the bathroom because you don't
have time to do both!

⁂

When people think you really want to
see what they blew out of their nose or
give you a Ziploc with the bugs that
were crawling in their kid's hair.

⁂

When you can sleep standing up.

When you beat all the *Jeopardy* contestants on the medical questions.

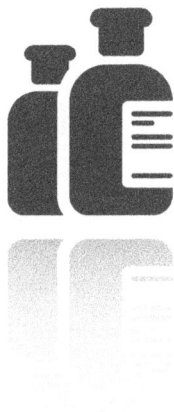

When you have frosted a cake with
a Ceftin spatula.

✳

When you fib about your occupation to
avoid the barrage of questions you
know you'll will be asked.

✳

When you dread the coming of
a full moon.

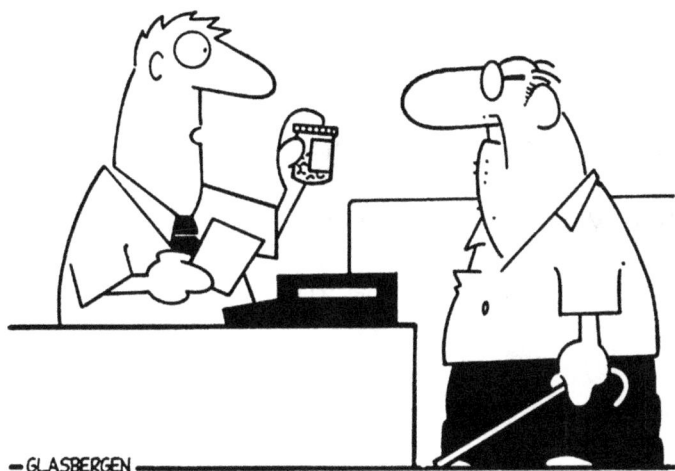

"Don't take these if you are nursing, pregnant or about to become pregnant."

When someone starts a question with,

"I realize you aren't a doctor but..."

✳

When you have pretty high standards

for what makes the perfect white coat,

label tape and pen.

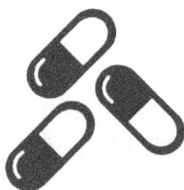

When you criticize medical stories on the news because they mispronounce the drug or disease.

When you consider foreign pharmacies
as tourist stops.

✺

When you can "hold it" for at least
eight hours.

✺

When you have the ability to forget
you are hungry.

When you estimate how long it will take everyone to leave the store when closing time is near.

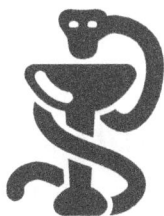

When the people you deal with have no problem waiting 45 minutes for a pizza delivery, yet expect their prescriptions to be filled in 10 minutes.

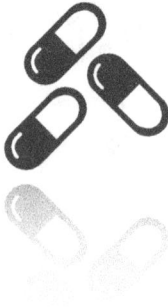

When you stand up and eat at home.
Usually over the sink.

✳

When you finish a meal before
everyone else at the table.

✳

When you think everyone takes too
long to decide anything.

When you've spilled pink amoxicillin
all over your white coat at one
point in your career.

❋

When you've cut or eaten your food
with a spatula!

❋

When you count pills in your sleep.

When you teach your children to count by fives using Skittles and a counting tray.

When you judge people
on whether they want
brand or generic.

When somebody says, "That long?" you
add five minutes to their wait time.

✳

When you never get sick unless you are
on vacation or it's your day off.

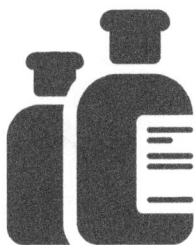

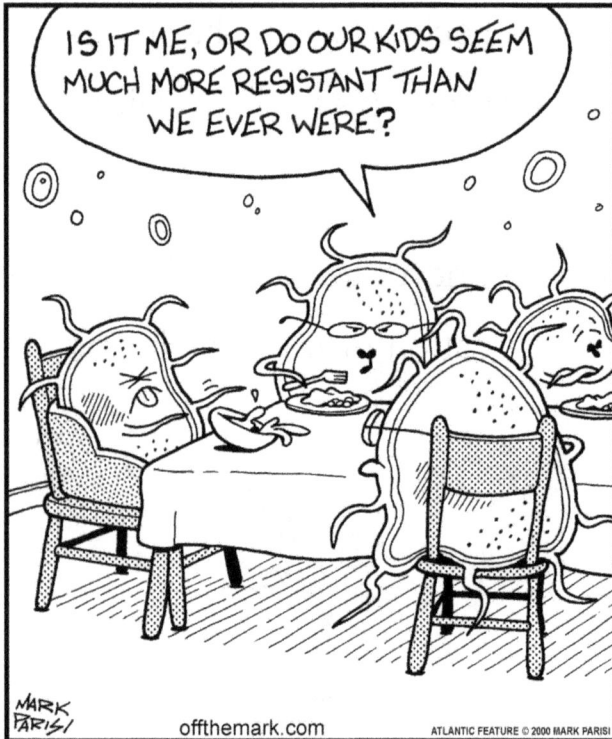

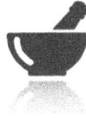

# 4

# Weird Science

In the retail environment, you can spend a lot of time "counting, pouring, licking and sticking." All that dispensing of meds leaves precious little time to dispense the sound, scientific advice you'd like to. Well, let's not waste all the cramming you did for mathematics, biology, chemistry and physics while studying for your pharmacy degree. Unlike most of the general public you serve, at least you'll get these jokes!

Two bacteria walk
into a hotel bar.
The bartender says,
"Get out. We don't serve
bacteria in this bar."
The bacteria reply,
"It's okay, we're staph."

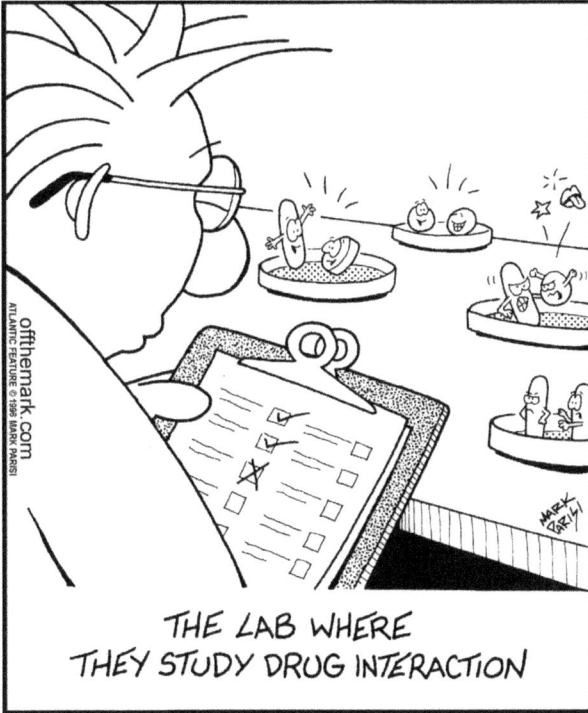

THE LAB WHERE
THEY STUDY DRUG INTERACTION

The guy who split
the atom is probably
thrilled that we use
"sliced bread"
as our measure
of greatness.

Isn't it ionic that oppositely charged atoms are attracted to each other?

*

If you're not part of the solution, you're either a solid or a gas.

*

Ar: The atomic symbol for Pirate.

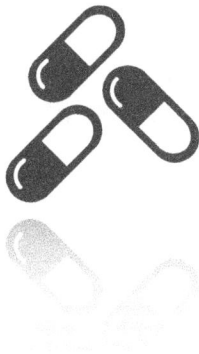

Went to a costume party the other day
as oxygen. I was in my element.

\*

I read Quantum Physics—but only
for the particles.

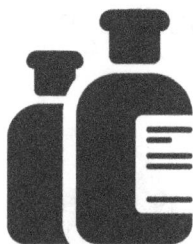

If Einstein hadn't
come up with the
Theory of Relativity,
someone else would have.
It was only a matter
of time.

At the lab today we mixed nitrous
oxide with mustard gas. We laughed
until we cried!

✳

I can't seem to be able to study
the model of an atom.
It's just too bohring.

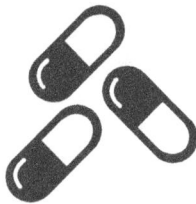

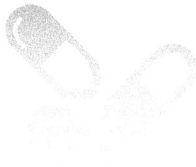

I thought I had all the angles covered,
but I still failed my geometry exam.

*

Biology: The only study in the world
that thinks division and multiplication
are the same thing.

I walked into
a room full of electrons—
it was so negative!

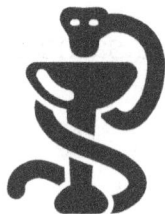

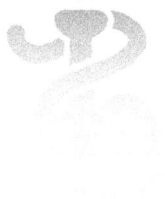

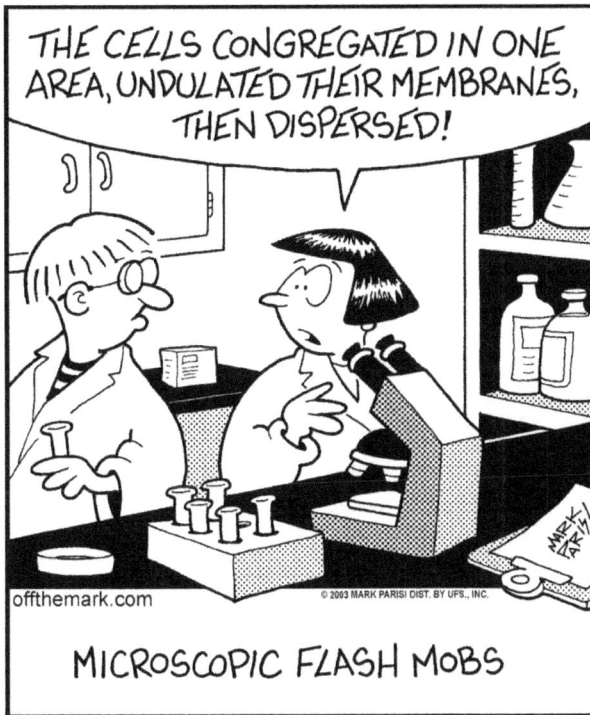

How often do I like to hear jokes about chemistry? Periodically.

✳

Can you tell me the formula for nitrogen oxide? NO.

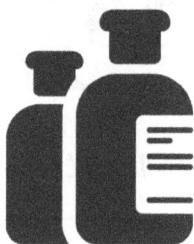

A woman approached me in town with a clipboard. "Are you happy with your energy supplier?" she asked. "I think so," I replied, "unless you've come up with a biological alternative to carbohydrates."

Carbon and boron walk into a bar.
Carbon turns to boron and says,
"If you were a bit more positive
you'd be just like me."

✳

A neutron walks into a bar and asks,
"How much for a beer?" The bartender
says, "For you, no charge."

Where does a chemistry professor
wash his dishes? In the zinc.

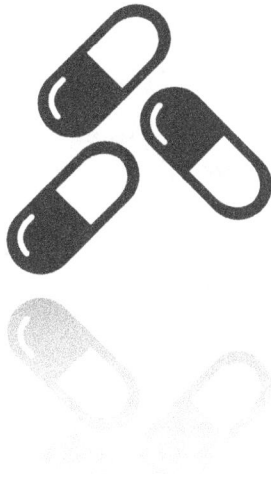

Asked to describe a Mobius strip,

I didn't know where to begin.

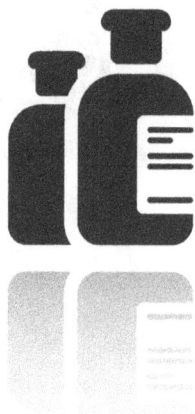

I went to a restaurant on the moon
the other day. The food was great,
but there wasn't really
any atmosphere.

❋

Biological terminology just keeps
getting cilia.

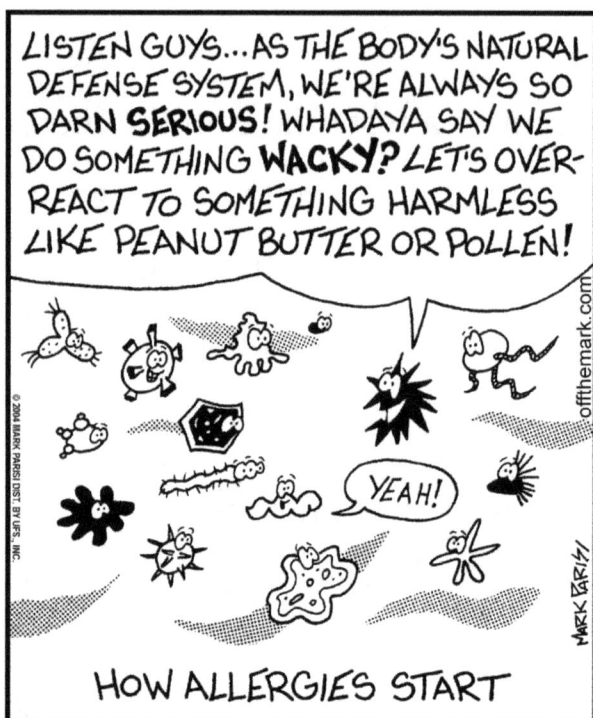

I was shown a molecular level diagram but couldn't see any of the particles. Maybe my eyesight is going, because I was looking right atom.

There's been some strange news about charged particles recently. I'm gonna' keep my ion it.

✳

I banged my neon the Periodic Table.

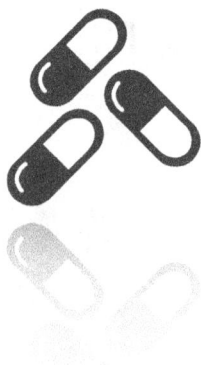

My biology teacher asked me, "Can you write a short essay on what would happen to somebody if their sudoriferous glands were removed?" I said, "Yeah, no sweat."

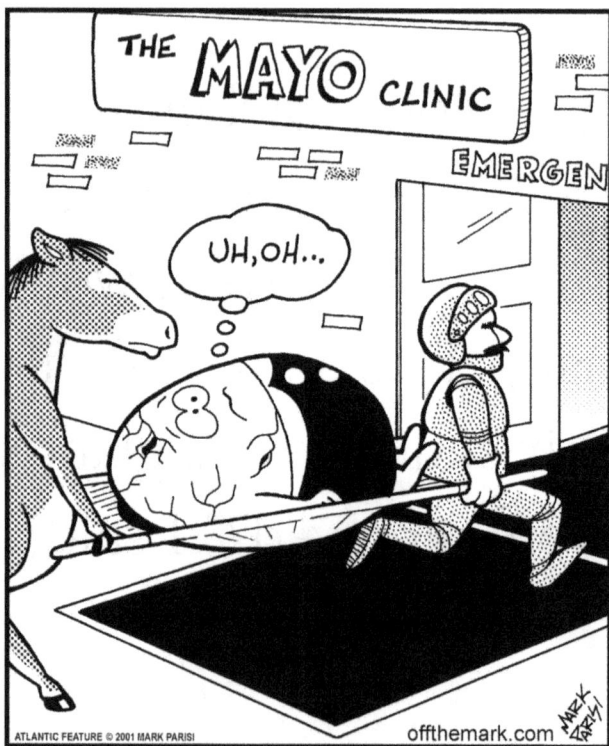

# 5

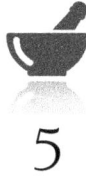

## Famous Pharmacists

Do you enjoy drinking a refreshing, cold soda on a hot summer day? Have you watched the classic film, *Murder on the Orient Express* or read "The Gift of the Magi"? (if not, I'd highly recommend you do.) Are you familiar with the 38th Vice President of the United States? (Hint: His boss was LBJ.) Do you think libraries benefit our society? Interestingly, all these questions have an answer in pharmacists! Take a look.

**Hubert Humphrey** (1911–1978): Serving under President Lyndon B. Johnson as the 38th Vice President of the United States. He earned his pharmacist license from the Capitol College of Pharmacy, Denver, Colorado, in 1931 and helped run his father's pharmacy, Humphrey Drug Company, for several years afterwards.

✳

**Benjamin Franklin** (1706–1790): One of the Founding Fathers of the United States. He created the first library in the country. Before he was a scientist, inventor, author, printer, postmaster and diplomat, he worked as a pharmacist dispensing medicines, herbs and various curatives in a neighborhood mercantile store.

**Agatha Christie** (1890–1976): The best-selling novelist of all time. Her books have sold over 4 billion copies! She qualified as a pharmacist in 1918 and during World War II worked in the pharmacy at University College Hospital, London, eventually putting her knowledge of poisons to good use in her post-war whodunits.

❋

**Wilbur Scoville** (1865–1942): American pharmacist and developer of The Scoville Organoleptic Test, now called the Scoville scale. Capsaicin, anyone?

**O. Henry** (1862–1910): Born William Sydney Porter, he was an American writer whose short stories are known for their clever-twist endings. Among his most famous stories is "The Gift of the Magi." O. Henry worked in his uncle's drugstore as a teenager and became a pharmacist at age 19.

**Friedrich Serturner** (1783–1841): German pharmacist who discovered morphine in 1804. In doing so, he became the first person to isolate the active ingredient of a medicinal plant or herb.

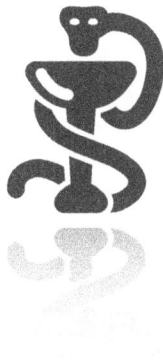

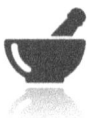

It isn't surprising
that pharmacists,
thirsty to create new
beverages for their
soda fountains,
invented some
of our favorite
soft drinks!

**John Pemberton** (1831–1888):

Inventor of Coca-Cola.

＊

**Charles Elmer Hires** (1851–1937):

Inventor of Hires Root Beer.

＊

**Charles Alderton** (1857–1941):

Inventor of Dr Pepper.

＊

**Caleb Bradham** (1867–1934):

Inventor of Pepsi Cola.

＊

**James Vernor** (1843–1927):

Inventor of Vernor's Ginger Ale.

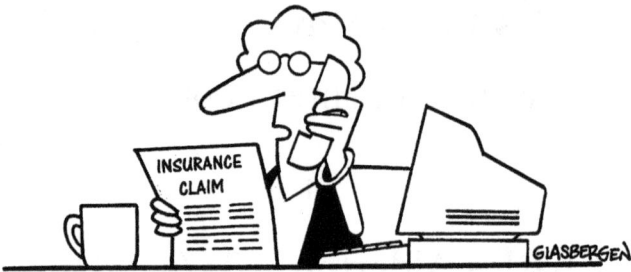

"Breakable bones, a tendency to bleed
when cut, vulnerability to germs and viruses.
These are all preexisting conditions."

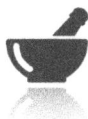

# 6

# Managed (*Don't*) Care

A physician once told me that it used to be called managed health care. "Then they took the health out of it and it became managed care!" Dealing with formularies isn't a terribly fulfilling part of your job (well, maybe it *is* terribly fulfilling), particularly when the insurance company increases a co-pay and the patient assumes it's at your discretion. But, if "nothing else" (which seems to be the new continuum of care model!) at least we get a few jokes out of all this foolishness.

Q. How is a hospital gown
like health insurance?

A. You're never covered
as much as you think
you are.

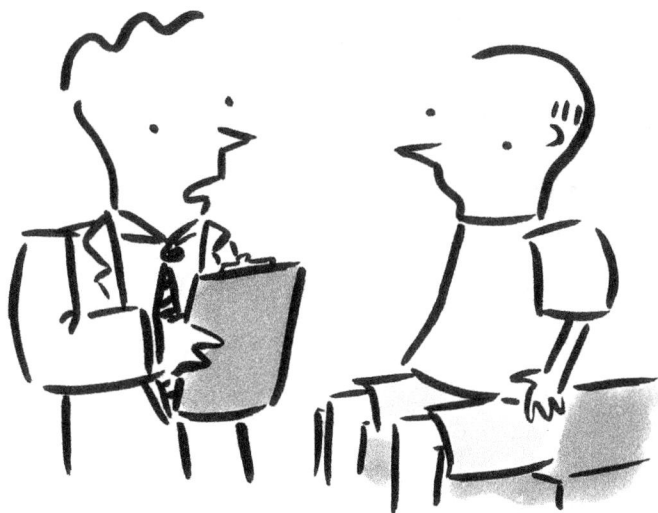

"I'm afraid neither daily apples nor prescription laughter is covered by your insurance."

If laughter truly is
the best medicine, health
plans would find a way
to charge for it.

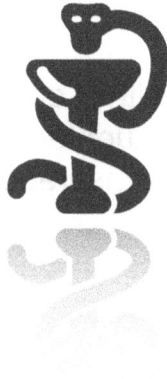

AN ELDERLY PATIENT in need of a heart transplant discussed his options with the doctor. "We have three possible donors," the doctor said. "One is a young, healthy athlete who died in an automobile accident. The second is a middle-aged businessman who never drank or smoked. The third is a managed care executive who died after working 30 years for a large insurance company." "I'll take the managed care executive's heart," said the patient. After a successful transplant, the doctor asked why he had chosen the donor he did. "It was easy," the patient replied. "I wanted a heart that hadn't been used."

*News Flash:* "Physicians working for a large care network have gone on strike. Officials, unclear on the doctors' demands, have sent a pharmacist to the picket line to read the signs."

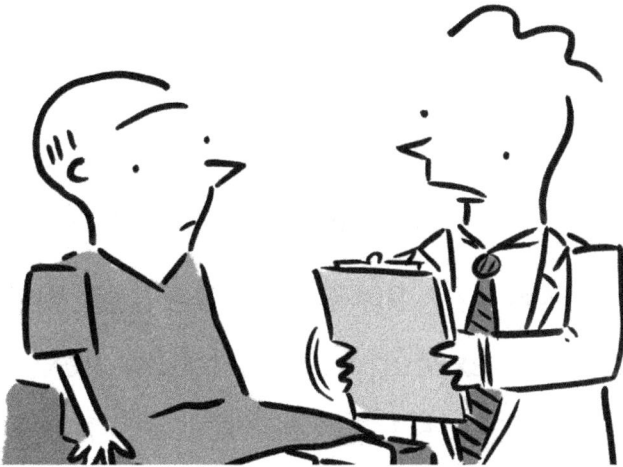

"We caught it early, but your insurance wants to let it go for a while and see what happens."

A DOCTOR IN a bar leans over to the guy next to him and says, "Wanna hear a managed care joke?" The guy replies, "Before you tell that joke, you should know something. I am 6 feet tall, weigh 200 pounds and I'm a managed care lawyer. The guy next to me is 6 feet, 2 inches, 225 pounds and he's a managed care executive. The fellow next to him is 6 feet 5 inches, 250 pounds and one of our second-level reviewers. Now, do you still wanna tell that joke?" The doctor says, "Nah, I don't want to have to explain it three times."

How can managed care executives make so many foolish mistakes in one day?  They get up early.

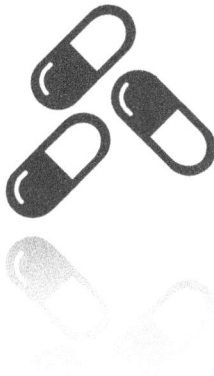

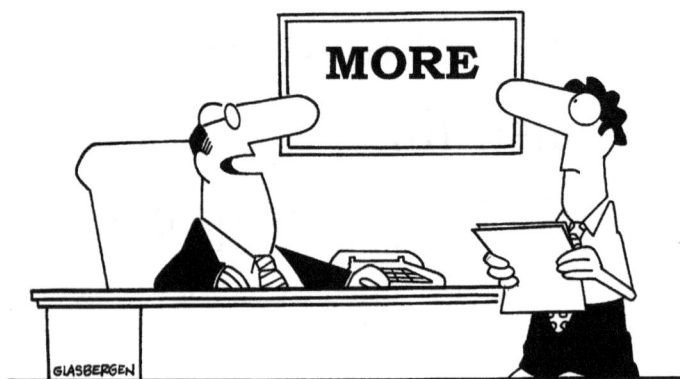

"That's our new mission statement."

# 7

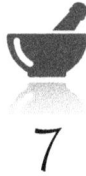

# Have I Got a Job for You!

In a recent Drug Topics salary survey, 75% of pharmacists report being satisfied, very satisfied or extremely satisfied with their positions. That's good news—but 67% feel their stress level has increased within the last year, due mostly to increased workload, lack of staff support and increased paperwork. Based on those results, the quips below may ring strangely true, but they do make for some pretty good one-liners!

The supermarket
pharmacy says: Must be
deadline oriented.
They mean: You'll be
six months behind
schedule on your
first day.

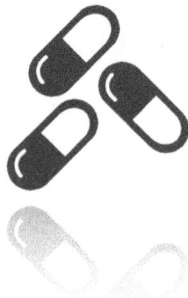

The big box pharmacy
says: Join our fast
paced team. They mean:
We have no time
to train you.

The chain drugstore says:
Seeking candidates with
a wide variety of
experience. They mean:
You'll need to replace
the two pharmacists
and one tech who
just left.

They all say:
Must be able to think on
your feet.

They all mean:
You won't be able to sit
down all day!

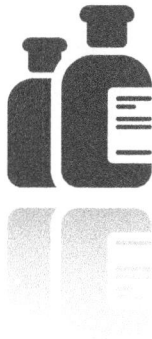

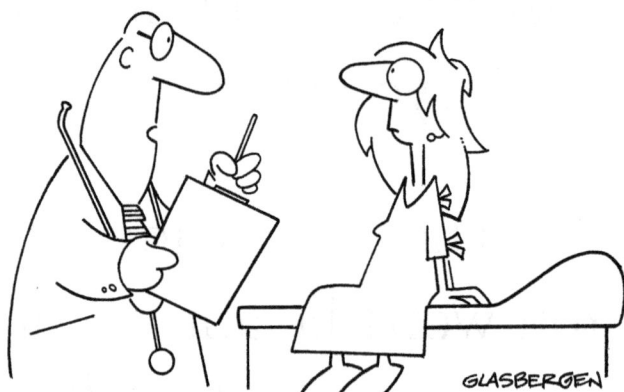

"You're in perfect health. Wait here while
I check what you should take for that."

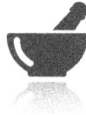

# 8

# Dr. Wizard of Oz

As a community pharmacist, I'm sure the majority of doctors you interact with are good, competent and "Dr. Oz-like." Still, you have your share of encounters with the "Dr. Wizard of Oz" types— those who aren't the capable physicians they appear to be, as evidenced by your "fixing" some of the issues they regularly cause (i.e., prescribing errors, paperwork problems, etc.). Regardless of their Oz or Wizard of Oz qualities, their profession does lend itself to some good old fashioned guffaws!

"Yeah, Doc, what's the news?" asked Fred, when his doctor called with the results. "I have some bad news and some really bad news," admitted the doctor. "The bad news is that you only have 24 hours to live." "Oh my," gasped Fred, sinking to his knees. "What could be worse news than that?" The doctor replied, "I couldn't get a hold of you yesterday."

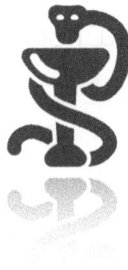

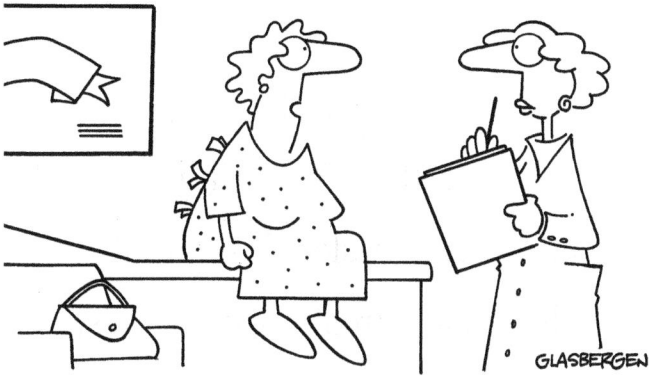

"That pill they advertise all the time on TV.
I'm not sure what it is, but I want it."

AN AMATEUR MAGICIAN accidentally turns his wife into a sofa and his two kids into recliners. He panics and tries every trick in the book to reverse it, but nothing works. In desperation, he takes them to the hospital. In the ER waiting room, the magician spends a sleepless night while the medical staff runs numerous tests on the unfortunate woman and children. Finally, a doctor comes out. "How is my family?" the magician asks worriedly. "Are they all right?" The doctor replies, "They're comfortable."

I went to the doctor the other day, and he told me, "I can't find a cause for your illness, though quite frankly I think it's the drinking." "Okay," I said, "I'll come back when you're sober."

*Dispense-sation*

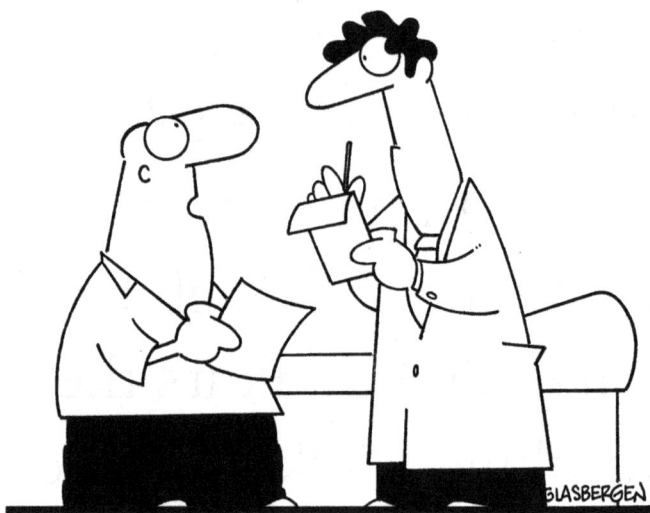

"Right now I take a blue pill, a purple pill, an orange pill, a white pill, and a yellow pill. I need you to prescribe a green pill to complete my collection."

I think my doctor likes me. She said
I have acute paranoia.

✳

"The doctor removed my left
ventricle and atrium," Tom said,
half-heartedly.

I went to the doctor because I was having trouble sleeping. "Hmm…," he said. "It sounds like insomnia." "Aw, c'mon Doc, I'm too tired for guessing games. Can't you just tell me what it is?"

I went to the doctor today and told her, "Every time I close my eyes I see pink striped tigers." "Have you seen a psychiatrist?" She asked. "No," I replied, "just pink striped tigers."

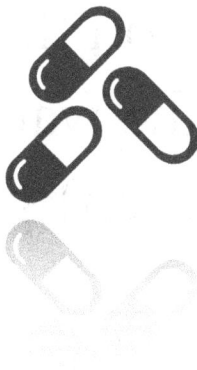

While having lunch at a restaurant, a doctor notices his waitress constantly scratching her hands. "Do you have eczema?" he asks.
"If it's not on the menu," says the waitress, "we haven't got it."

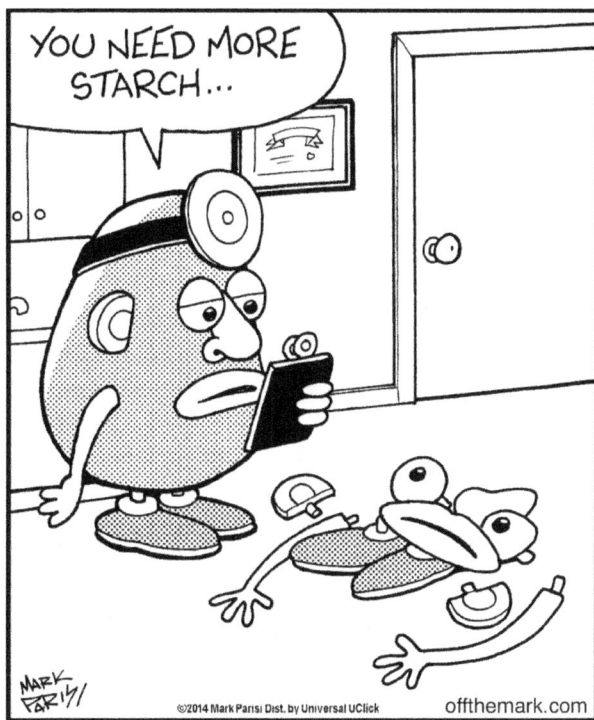

As a doctor and chef, it's not often that my skills are required all at once. Today was an exception. In preparing dinner, I had to cure the ham.

The doctor told me I'm partially deaf, which was difficult to hear.

✳

Doctor: "How are you feeling today?"

Patient: "With my hands mainly, same as yesterday."

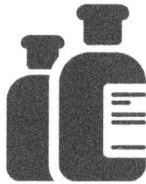

The inventor of the adjective is seriously ill in the hospital.
Doctors have been unable to describe his condition.

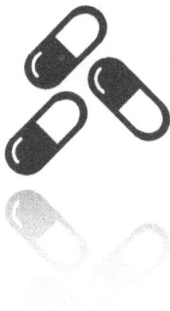

I WENT TO see the doctor because of an outbreak of itchy, weeping sores all over my body. She examined me, prescribed a bottle of pills and said, "Just follow the instructions and you should be back to normal within ten days." For two weeks now I've been keeping them away from direct sunlight and out of reach of young children, and if anything, my condition has gotten worse.

# Prescriptions

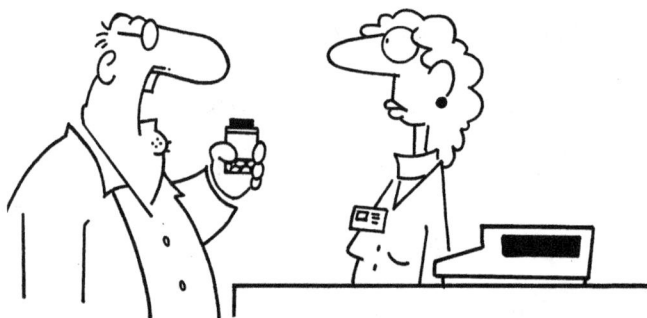

"I've been taking this medication for 50 years and I'm going to sue! The side effects made me wrinkled, fat and bald!"

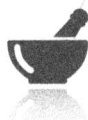

# 9

# Mortar and Pests

Serving patients who appreciate your advice and counsel make up for the few who don't. Said another way, some patients test your patience more than others! Below is an attempt—in a spirit of good cheer—to articulate what you *may* be thinking (sometimes?) when dealing with them.

If you gave him a penny for his
thoughts, you'd get change.

❖

If he had another brain,
it would be lonely.

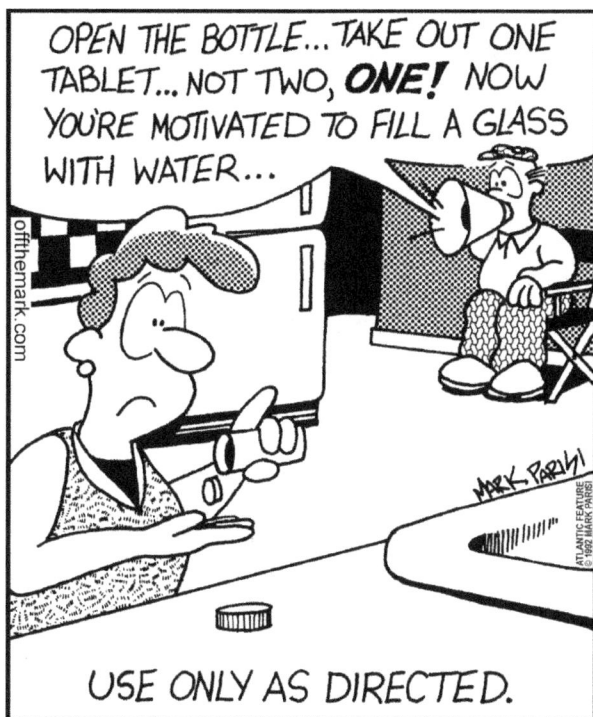

As smart as bait.

✻

Proof that evolution can
go in reverse.

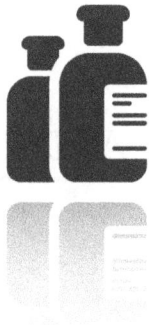

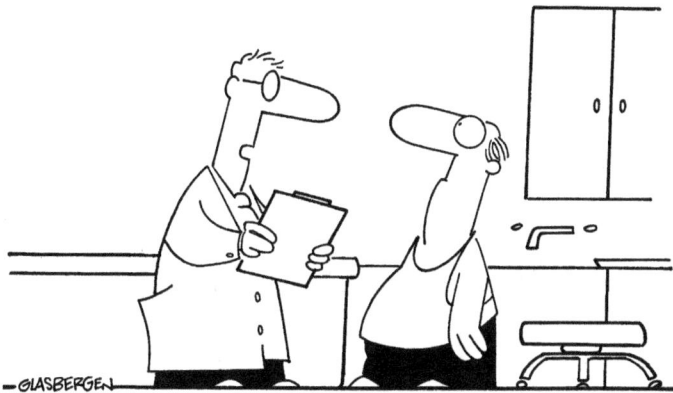

"No, HDL and LDL were not the robots in Star Wars."

When she opens her mouth, it's only to change feet.

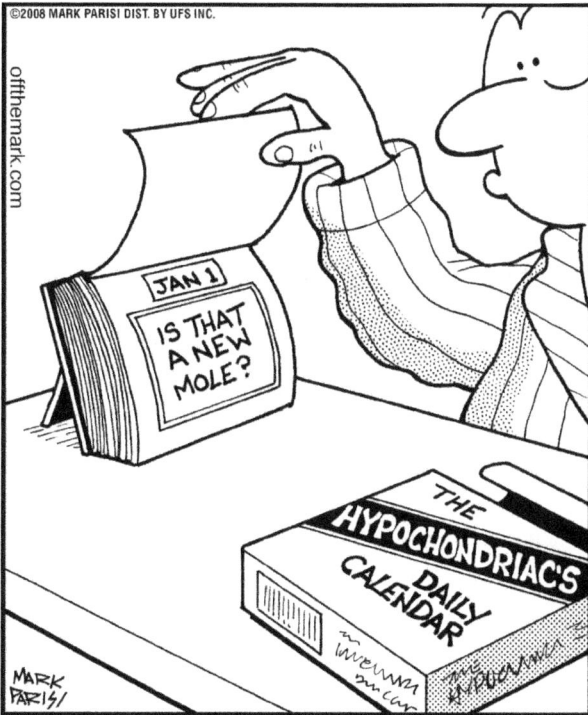

Some drink from the
fountain of knowledge;
he only gargles.

If you stand close enough to him,
you can hear the ocean.

⁕

Too much yardage between the
goalposts.

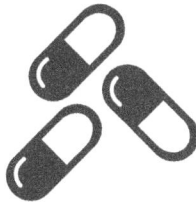

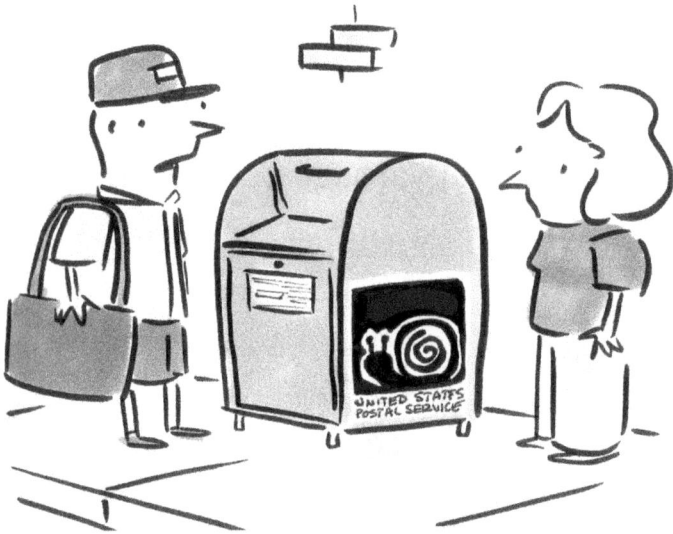

"We finally decided to just embrace it."

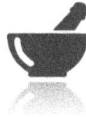

# 10

# Wait a Minute, Mr. Postman

*Neither snow, nor rain, nor heat, nor gloom of night stays these courageous couriers from the swift completion of delivering...**the mail order prescriptions**.*

Ok, I took some liberty with that saying —but why not? PBMs pushing mandatory mail order pharmacy are not looking out for the community pharmacist. Of course, I don't blame the Post Office for their participation, but I can't pass up this golden opportunity to use them as the punch line! And, somewhat seriously, these jokes should give you not only a chuckle but a glimmer of hope too!

One good thing about the
Post Office. It's over
200 years old, yet
it's never been hindered
by progress.

If you want to make sure somebody gets what's coming to 'em, for goodness sake—don't mail it!

❋

My Post Office uses four checkouts. Unless it's really busy— then they use one.

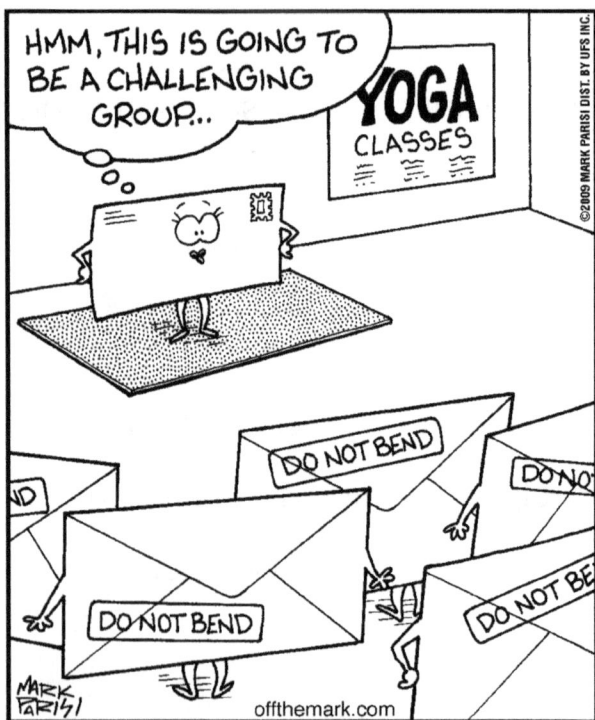

I remember when
postal workers started a
slow-down strike
for a pay raise.
They had to call it off—
nobody noticed.

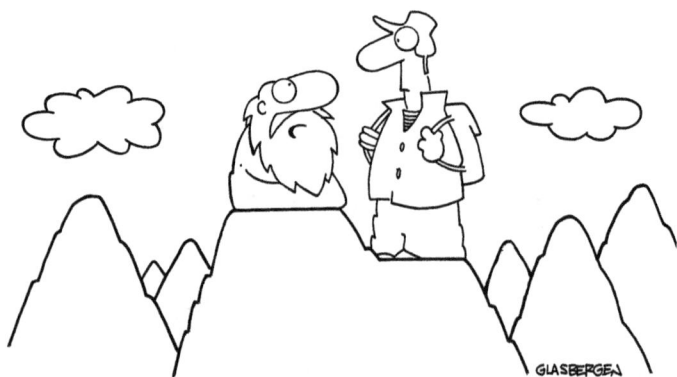

"No, I can't tell you the meaning of life.
I only came up here to avoid carbs."

# 11

# The Wise Pharmacist Says…

*Be as smart as you can, but remember that it is always better to be wise than to be smart.*

–Alan Alda

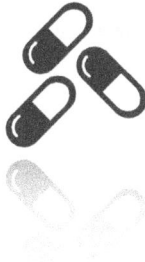

The sooner you fall behind, the more time you'll have to catch up.

The severity of the itch is
proportional to the reach.

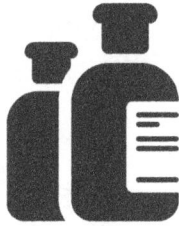

If you think health
care is expensive now,
imagine how expensive
it will be when
it's "free."

The problem with being an
independent pharmacy owner
is when you do something wrong
you're fined, and when you do
something right, you're taxed!

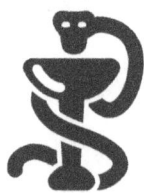

Being a pharmacist
is a good job if
you're on a diet.

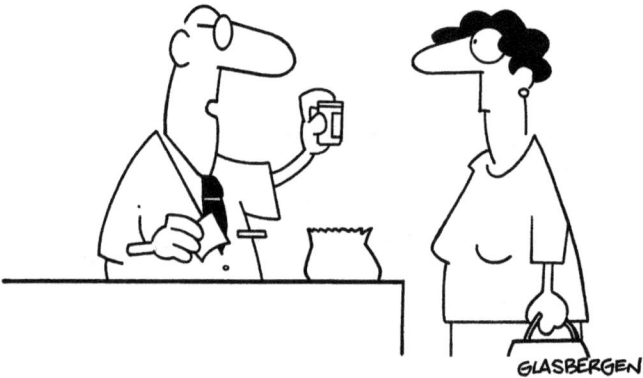

"This is one of those new miracle drugs.
If you can afford it, it's a miracle."

Without hard
work, nothing
grows but
shrinkage.

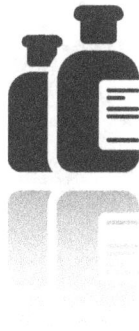

Dispensing errors are stepping stones to
learning and a criminal conviction.

✳

Opportunity does not knock;
it walks straight in with a nine-item
script at 8:55 p.m.

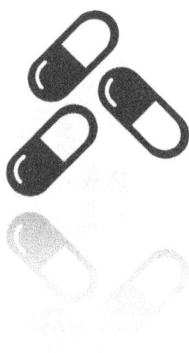

I think the difference between a young, new owner of an independent pharmacy and a savings bond is that eventually, one of them matures and earns money.

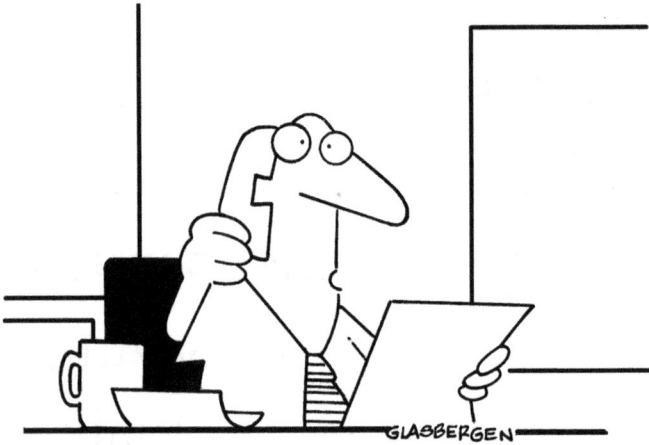

"Our legal department wants us to download their new software. It translates gobbledygook to mumbo jumbo."

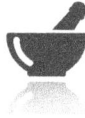

# 12

# Lowering the Bar

The fine print in a PBM contract. Compliance with HIPPA. A lawsuit. The common denominator? Lawyers. A population you're sometimes forced to deal with whose members don't add much, if anything, to your bottom line or peace of mind. Well, if you can't beat them, at least "enjoin" them (sort of!) with some humor. (Legal disclaimer: These jokes are not intended to diagnose, treat, cure or prevent any disease.)

99% of lawyers give the rest
a bad name.

✻

A lawyer is a person who writes a
10,000-word PBM contract and
calls it a brief.

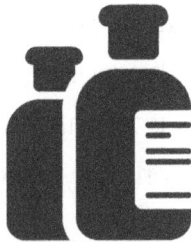

THREE MEN WERE traveling together: a preacher, a cowboy and a lawyer. It was getting late and they needed a place to sleep. At last, they came across a farm and asked the farmer if they could spend the night. "That's fine," he said, "but my guest room is only big enough for two people. One of you will have to sleep in the barn." The preacher said, "I don't mind sleeping with God's creatures. I will take the barn." About an hour later, there was a knock at the guest room door and there stood the preacher. "I can't stand the smell from that cow in there anymore. I'm sorry, but I'm going to have to sleep in the guest room." "That's okay," said the cowboy, "I'll sleep in the barn." About an hour later, there was a knock at the guest room door and there stood the cowboy. "There's a chicken in the barn that won't stop clucking! I'm sorry, but I'm going to have to sleep in the guest room." "Well, I guess that leaves me," said the lawyer. So he went to sleep in the barn. About an hour later, there was a knock at the guest room door, and there stood the chicken and the cow.

Lawyer: "You seem to be quite a bit smarter than the average witness from your background."

Witness: "Why thank you. If I wasn't under oath, I could return the compliment."

I asked my lawyer
how he sleeps at night.
"First I lie on one side,"
he said, "and then I lie
on the other."

What's wrong with lawyer jokes? Lawyers don't think they're funny and nobody else thinks they're jokes.

✳

Cross a librarian and a lawyer and what do you get? All the information you want, except you can't understand it.

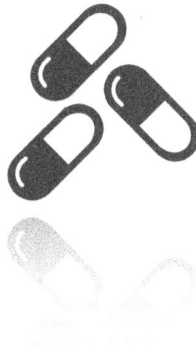

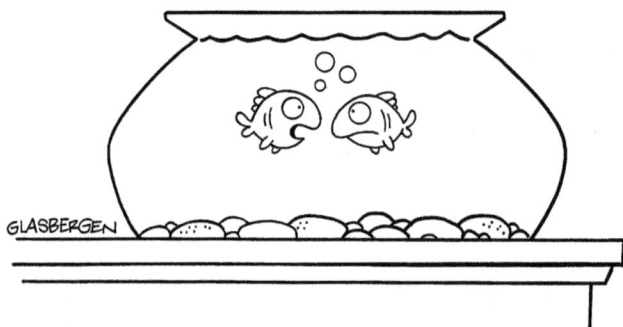

"When do they take us out to go to the bathroom? I don't think I can hold it much longer!"

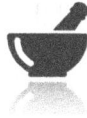

# 13

# Irritable Jowl Syndrome

*n. a widespread dropping of the jaw, often associated with people who don't have the slightest clue what a retail pharmacist's day is really like, upon learning that going to the bathroom falls outside the scope of the job.*

In the spirit of laughing at what can be frustrating, with bathroom breaks a challenge on a busy retail day, here are a few jokes "to go."

DRIVING ACROSS MICHIGAN, a man needed to use a bathroom and pulled into a rest stop. Once inside, he entered the stall, sat down and was surprised to hear someone in the next stall ask, "So how ya doing?" The man gulped, cleared his throat and nervously said, "Uh... I'm fine." The same voice then asked, "So where are you headed?" Again the man, a little nervous, answered, "Uh... I'm heading east." Then another question. "So what have you been up to?" "Not much, I'm actually on a business trip," the man replied. Suddenly, the stranger in the next stall abruptly said, "Look, I'm going to have to call you back. Some strange guy in the next stall thinks I'm talking to him."

Somebody broke into the police station and stole the only toilet in the building. The cops are anxious to apprehend the perpetrator, but they have nothing to go on.

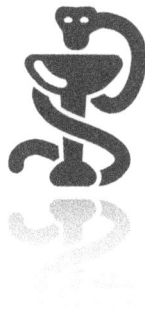

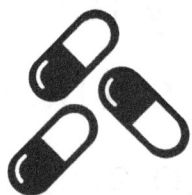

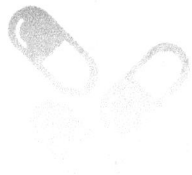

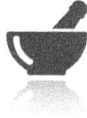

# 14

# All Kidding Aside

*Wherever the art of medicine is loved,
there is also a love of humanity.*
–Hippocrates

I hope this book has achieved what it set out to do—create an occasion (or dare I say an excuse) for you to slow down, put your feet up and laugh at some of the things you regularly deal with as a retail pharmacist.

The lightheartedness of the material by no means diminishes the seriousness of your work. The contribution your profession has made to the health care system is significant. The community pharmacist is among the most accessible and trusted sources of healthcare. You counsel on everything from head lice to hemorrhoids and provide patients with services like MTM, blood pressure checks, cholesterol and osteoporosis screenings, tobacco cessation programs, glucose screenings, diabetes education, weight loss counseling, compounding and specialty services and life-saving immunizations.

Beyond the walls of the retail pharmacy, you often practice in a wide range of other settings during your career, including hospitals, health centers and long-term-care facilities. You work in government and in the pharmaceutical industry as well as provide support for hospice, home-care environments and community health fairs.

Thankfully, your efforts, particularly as a "front line" retail pharmacist, have not gone unrecognized or unappreciated by those you care about most. As evidenced by the Gallup Poll, you are perennially ranked by your patients as one of the most trusted professionals in America. Said another way, you are indispensable!

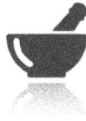

# Acknowledgments

To pharmacists everywhere—as much as you are the intended recipients of this book, you are also the contributors. You've shared what life as a pharmacist is like through personal interactions and professional discussions, as well as through your insightful (and often humorous) blogs, articles and other social media postings. Thanks for making this book possible.

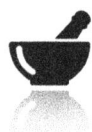

www.ingramcontent.com/pod-product-compliance
Lightning Source LLC
Chambersburg PA
CBHW060302050426
42448CB00009B/1720